The Art of Skipping

Mastering the Fundamentals of Jump Rope for Fitness, Fun, and Competition

By

Alex Lenero

Kindle Edition

Contents

Introduction

Jump rope has been a beloved pastime for generations, enjoyed by children and adults alike. But despite its simple appearance, jump rope is a dynamic and challenging sport that requires skill, coordination, and endurance. In "The Art of Skipping," we explore the rich history of jump rope and its many benefits, from improved cardiovascular health to increased mental focus. Whether you're a beginner or an experienced jumper, this book provides everything you need to know to master the art of skipping.

History of Jump Rope

Jump rope has a long and fascinating history, with roots that can be traced back to ancient civilizations. Evidence of rope jumping can be found in Egyptian hieroglyphics, and the Chinese and Greeks also used rope jumping as a form of exercise and entertainment.

In the 19th century, jump rope became a popular pastime for children in Europe and the United States, often played in schoolyards and streets. The first recorded jump rope competitions were held in the 1930s, and the sport continued to grow in popularity over the next several decades.

Jump rope has since evolved into a highly competitive sport, with events and competitions held around the world. From individual and team events to freestyle and speed jumping, there are many different styles of jump rope for competitors to master. Today, jump rope is recognized as a fun and effective form of exercise enjoyed by people of all ages and fitness levels.

Benefits of Jump Rope

Jump rope provides a wide range of physical and mental benefits, making it an excellent form of exercise for people of all ages and fitness levels. Some of the benefits of jump rope include:

umping rope is a highly effective and beneficial exercise that provides a wide range of physical and mental benefits. Here are 10 benefits of jump rope:

1. Improves cardiovascular health: Jumping rope is a high-intensity aerobic exercise that helps to improve your heart health and cardiovascular endurance.

2. Burns calories: Jumping rope is an excellent way to burn calories and lose weight. It can burn up to 10 calories per minute, making it one of the most efficient calorie-burning exercises.

3. Builds stamina: Regular jump rope practice can help to build your stamina and endurance, allowing you to perform physical activities for longer periods of time.

4. Tones muscles: Jumping rope engages the muscles in your legs, core, and upper body, helping to tone and strengthen them over time.

5. Increases coordination and balance: Jumping rope requires coordination and balance, which can improve over time with regular practice.

6. Enhances bone density: Jumping rope is a weight-bearing exercise that can help to strengthen your bones and reduce the risk of osteoporosis.

7. Reduces stress: Jumping rope is a great stress-relieving exercise that can help to release endorphins and reduce feelings of anxiety and depression.

8. Improves agility and speed: Jumping rope requires quick movements and reflexes, which can help to improve your agility and speed.

9. Enhances cognitive function: Jumping rope requires concentration and focus, which can enhance cognitive function and improve brain health.

10. Boosts overall fitness: Jumping rope is a highly effective exercise that can improve your overall fitness level, including strength, endurance, flexibility, and cardiovascular health.

When it comes to practicing jump rope, it is generally better to practice on a flat and even surface like concrete, asphalt, or a gym floor. Grass can be uneven and bumpy, which can make it difficult to maintain a consistent jumping rhythm and can also increase the risk of tripping and falling. Additionally, jumping on grass can cause the rope to get tangled or caught in the grass, which can be frustrating and disrupt your workout.

That being said, if you have joint pain or other issues that make it uncomfortable to jump on a hard surface, grass can provide some cushioning and reduce the impact on your joints. In this case, it may be better to use a thicker, heavier jump rope that doesn't tangle as easily and to jump in an area of the grass that is as flat and even as possible.

Ultimately, the choice of surface depends on personal preference and individual circumstances. If you have access to a gym or a flat, even surface like a driveway or parking lot, that would be the ideal surface to practice jump rope. If you don't have access to such surfaces, grass can be a suitable alternative if you take the necessary precautions and choose the right type of rope.

Setting Goals

Setting goals is an important part of any exercise program, including jump rope. Goals provide direction, motivation, and a way to track progress. When setting goals for jump rope, consider the following tips:

1. Be Specific: Set specific, measurable, and achievable goals. For example, "I want to be able to do 50 double unders in a row" is a specific goal, while "I want to get better at jump rope" is not.

2. Make Them Realistic: Make sure your goals are realistic and achievable within a specific timeframe. It's important to challenge yourself, but setting unrealistic goals can lead to disappointment and discourage you from continuing.

3. Write Them Down: Writing down your goals helps to make them more concrete and provides a visual reminder of what you're working towards.

4. Track Progress: Keep track of your progress toward your goals and celebrate your achievements along the way. This will help to keep you motivated and on track.

5. Be Flexible: Life is unpredictable, and sometimes goals may need to be adjusted. Be flexible and willing to adjust your goals as needed, but continue to work towards your overall vision.

Remember, the most important thing is to have fun and enjoy the process. Jump rope is a fun and dynamic sport, and setting goals is just one way to make the most of your jumping experience.

Getting Started

Getting started with jump rope can be intimidating, but with the right tools and some practice, anyone can learn to skip. Here are some tips to help you get started:

1. Choose the Right Rope: Selecting the right rope is an important part of getting started with jump rope. Consider the length, weight, and material of the rope when making your selection.

2. Learn the Basic Techniques: Start by learning the basic jump rope techniques, including the basic jump, alternating feet, and jumping with a bouncy rhythm.

3. Warm-Up and Stretch: Always warm up and stretch before jumping to prevent injury. This can include light cardio, such as jogging or jumping jacks, and stretching the muscles used in jumping.

4. Practice Regularly: Consistent practice is key to improving your jump rope skills. Aim to practice for at least 10-15 minutes each day, gradually increasing the length and intensity of your sessions as you get stronger.

5. Seek Out Resources: There are many resources available to help you get started with jump rope, including books, videos, and online tutorials. Take advantage of these resources to learn new techniques and get tips and tricks from more experienced jumpers.

6. Have Fun: Remember, jump rope is supposed to be fun! Don't get discouraged if you make mistakes or struggle at first. With practice and

patience, you'll get better, and before you know it, you'll be skipping like a pro

Here are 10 of the best jump rope brands based on their quality, durability, and customer reviews:

1. RX Smart Gear: RX Smart Gear jump ropes are made with high-quality materials and come in a variety of sizes and styles to suit different needs and preferences.

2. Crossrope: Crossrope is a popular jump rope brand that offers a range of different weighted ropes for different fitness levels and goals.

3. Rogue Fitness: Rogue Fitness is a well-known fitness equipment brand that also makes high-quality jump ropes for various types of workouts.

4. WOD Nation: WOD Nation makes a variety of jump ropes for different levels of skill and fitness, including speed ropes and weighted ropes.

5. EliteSRS: EliteSRS jump ropes are designed for athletes and fitness enthusiasts who want a durable and high-performing rope for their workouts.

6. King Athletic: King Athletic makes high-quality jump ropes for various types of workouts, including cardio, CrossFit, and boxing.

7. Survival and Cross: Survival and Cross makes affordable jump ropes that are durable and suitable for various types of fitness activities.

8. Sonic Boom: Sonic Boom jump ropes are designed to be fast, smooth, and durable, making them a popular choice among athletes and fitness enthusiasts.

9. Benvo: Benvo jump ropes are affordable and come in a range of different colors and styles, making them a popular choice for beginners.

10. GoxRunx: GoxRunx jump ropes are designed for speed and durability, making them a great option for high-intensity workouts and cardio training.

Here are some step-by-step instructions for how to start skipping:

1. Get a jump rope: You can purchase a jump rope at most sporting goods stores, or online. Make sure to choose a rope that is appropriate for your height.

2. Wear appropriate footwear: Make sure to wear comfortable and supportive sneakers or shoes. This will help to prevent any injuries.

3. Choose a suitable surface: It's best to skip on a surface that is flat, level and has some cushioning, such as a rubber mat, a wooden floor or a grassy area.

4. Adjust the rope length: Hold the jump rope by the handles and stand on the center of the rope with both feet. The handles should reach up to your armpits. If the rope is too long, you can adjust it by tying knots on the ends or cutting it with scissors.

5. Begin with basic jumps: Start by practicing basic jumps, also known as single unders. Swing the rope over your head and jump over it with both feet at the same time. As you land, make sure to keep your feet together and your knees slightly bent.

6. Practice regularly: Set aside a few minutes each day to practice skipping. Start with short sessions of a few minutes, and gradually increase the time as you become more comfortable and confident.

7. Experiment with different styles: Once you've mastered the basic jump, you can experiment with different styles of skipping, such as double unders, criss-cross jumps, and side swings. Watch online tutorials or ask for tips from more experienced skippers to learn these more advanced techniques.

Remember to warm up before you start skipping to prevent any injuries, and don't push yourself too hard too soon

Choosing the Right Rope

Choosing the right jump rope is an important part of getting started with jump rope. Consider the following factors when making your selection:

1. Length: The length of the rope should be adjusted to your height. To determine the correct length, stand on the center of the rope with your arms extended straight up, and the handles should reach your armpits.

2. Weight: Jump ropes come in different weights, with lighter ropes being easier to control and heavier ropes providing more resistance. Consider your skill level and the type of jumping you plan to do when selecting the weight of your rope.

3. Material: Jump ropes can be made of a variety of materials, including plastic, leather, and cable. Plastic ropes are the most affordable and lightweight, while cable ropes are more durable and provide more resistance.

4. Handles: Look for handles that are comfortable to grip and easy to hold. Some handles are coated in foam, while others have a textured surface to prevent slippage.

5. Adjustability: Consider whether the rope is adjustable, as this allows you to fine-tune the length of the rope to your specific needs.

6. Purpose: If you plan to use your jump rope for fitness, competition, or tricks, consider the specific needs of each activity when making your selection.

Basic Techniques

Mastering the basic techniques of jump rope is the foundation of becoming a skilled jumper. Here are some of the most important basic techniques to learn:

1. Basic Jump: This is the most basic jump, where you jump with both feet over the rope as it swings under your feet.

2. Alternating Feet: This technique involves jumping with one foot at a time, alternating feet as the rope swings under you.

3. Bouncy Rhythm: This technique involves jumping with a bouncy rhythm, using your arms and legs to generate momentum and keep the rope moving.

4. Swing: This technique involves swinging the rope over your head and under your feet, using a smooth and consistent motion to keep the rope moving.

5. Timing: Timing is an important part of jump rope, and involves jumping at the right moment to clear the rope as it swings under your feet.

Warm-Up and Stretching

Warming up and stretching before jump rope is an important part of preventing injury and ensuring a safe and effective workout. Here are some tips for warming up and stretching before jump rope:

1. Light Cardio: Start with 5-10 minutes of light cardio, such as jogging or jumping jacks, to get your heart rate up and warm up your muscles.

2. Dynamic Stretching: Dynamic stretching involves moving your muscles through a full range of motion, helping to prepare your body for the demands of jump rope. Examples of dynamic stretching include leg swings, high knees, and butt kicks.

3. Targeted Stretching: Focus on stretching the muscles used in jump rope, including the calf muscles, quadriceps, hamstrings, and hips. Hold each stretch for 15-30 seconds, and repeat each stretch 2-3 times.

4. Cool Down: After your jump rope session, be sure to cool down and stretch again to help prevent muscle soreness and stiffness.

Advanced Techniques

Once you've mastered the basic techniques of jump rope, it's time to move on to more advanced techniques. Here are some of the most popular advanced techniques to explore:

1. Double Unders: This technique involves jumping with both feet and swinging the rope under your feet twice in one jump.

2. Crosses: This technique involves crossing the rope in front of and behind your feet as you jump, creating a more dynamic and challenging jumping experience.

3. Speed Skipping: This technique involves jumping as quickly as possible, using a bouncy rhythm and powerful arm movements to keep the rope moving.

4. Tricks and Combinations: Jump rope tricks and combinations involve adding flips, spins, and other movements to your jumping, creating a more dynamic and entertaining experience.

5. Freestyle Jumping: Freestyle jumping involves incorporating music, creative movements, and tricks into your jumping, creating a unique and personalized performance.

Double Unders Crosses

Double unders and crosses are advanced jump rope techniques that take time and practice to master. Here's a brief overview of each technique:

1. Double Unders: Double unders are a challenging technique that involves jumping with both feet and swinging the rope under your feet twice in one jump. To perform double unders, you'll need to generate enough speed and momentum with your arms and legs to keep the rope moving quickly. Start by practicing double unders slowly and gradually increasing your speed as you become more comfortable with the technique.

2. Crosses: Crosses involve crossing the rope in front of and behind your feet as you jump, creating a more dynamic and challenging jumping experience. To perform crosses, you'll need to coordinate your arm movements with your jumping and have good timing to avoid tripping on the rope. Start by practicing crosses slowly and gradually increasing your speed as you become more comfortable with the technique.

Both double unders and crosses are advanced techniques that require a good foundation of basic jumping skills and endurance. With practice and patience, you'll be able to master these techniques and take your jumping to the next level.

Speed Skipping

Speed skipping is an advanced jump rope technique that involves jumping as quickly as possible, using a bouncy rhythm and powerful arm movements to keep the rope moving. Speed skipping is a high-intensity workout that can improve cardiovascular health and increase endurance. Here are some tips to help you get started with speed skipping:

1. Warm-Up: Start with a thorough warm-up, including light cardio and dynamic stretching, to prepare your body for the demands of speed skipping.

2. Bouncy Rhythm: Use a bouncy rhythm to generate momentum and keep the rope moving quickly. Move your arms and legs in a coordinated and fluid motion to maintain speed and control.

3. Timing: Good timing is key to speed skipping, as you'll need to jump at the right moment to clear the rope as it swings under your feet. Start by practicing at a slower speed and gradually increasing your speed as you become more comfortable with the technique.

4. Endurance: Speed skipping is a high-intensity workout that requires good endurance. Gradually increase the length and intensity of your speed skipping sessions, taking breaks as needed to avoid fatigue.

5. Practice Regularly: Regular practice is the key to improving your speed skipping skills. Aim to practice for at least 10-15 minutes each day, gradually increasing the length and intensity of your sessions as you get stronger.

Speed skipping is an advanced technique that requires time and practice to master. With patience and dedication, you'll soon be able to perform speed skipping with ease and confidence.

Tricks and Combinations

Jump rope tricks and combinations add an element of creativity and entertainment to your jumping, making it a fun and dynamic sport. Here are some popular tricks and combinations to try:

1. Flips: This trick involves flipping the rope over your head and catching it on the other side, adding a dynamic and challenging element to your jumping.

2. Spins: This trick involves spinning the rope around your body, either by swinging it in a circular motion or by jumping over it as it spins.

3. Jumps with Leg Swings: This combination involves adding leg swings to your jumping, either by kicking your legs out to the side or by crossing them in front of or behind your body.

4. Jumps with Arm Swings: This combination involves adding arm swings to your jumping, either by swinging your arms in a circular motion or by crossing them in front of or behind your body.

5. Jumps with Knee Lifts: This combination involves adding knee lifts to your jumping, either by lifting your knees to your chest or by alternating knees with each jump.

Jump rope tricks and combinations require coordination, timing, and practice to master. Start with simple tricks and combinations, and gradually add more complex elements as you become more comfortable with your jumping. Remember, the most important thing is to have fun and enjoy the process!

Training and Conditioning

Training and conditioning are important components of improving your jump rope skills and reaching your goals. Here are some tips for effective training and conditioning:

1. Warm-Up and Stretch: Always warm up and stretch before jumping to prevent injury and ensure a safe and effective workout.

2. Set Goals: Set specific, achievable goals for your jump rope training and use these goals to guide your workouts and track your progress.

3. Practice Regularly: Consistent practice is key to improving your jump rope skills. Aim to practice for at least 10-15 minutes each day, gradually increasing the length and intensity of your sessions as you get stronger.

4. Incorporate Variety: Mix up your jump rope workouts to keep them interesting and prevent boredom. Try different techniques, combinations, and tricks, and incorporate other forms of exercise into your routine, such as strength training and cardio.

5. Focus on Technique: Good technique is key to improving your jump rope skills and preventing injury. Take the time to focus on proper form and technique during your workouts, and seek out feedback and tips from more experienced jumpers.

6. Listen to Your Body: Jump rope is a high-impact activity, and it's important to listen to your body and avoid overtraining. Take breaks as needed, and be mindful of any signs of injury or fatigue.

Training and conditioning are an important part of jump rope, and with patience and dedication, you'll be able to achieve your goals and reach your full potential as a jumper.

Building Endurance

Building endurance is an important part of jump rope and requires consistent practice and a gradual increase in intensity. Here are some tips for building endurance:

1. Start Slow: Start with short jump rope sessions and gradually increase the length and intensity of your workouts as you get stronger.

2. Incorporate Intervals: Interval training, where you alternate periods of high-intensity jumping with periods of rest or light jumping, can help to build endurance and improve cardiovascular health.

3. Focus on Proper Form: Good technique is key to building endurance and avoiding injury. Focus on proper form and technique during your workouts, and seek out feedback and tips from more experienced jumpers.

4. Mix Up Your Workouts: Incorporating variety into your jump rope workouts can help to prevent boredom and keep you motivated. Try different techniques, combinations, and tricks, and incorporate other forms of exercise into your routine, such as strength training and cardio.

5. Set Goals: Set specific, achievable goals for your jump rope training, and use these goals to guide your workouts and track your progress.

6. Listen to Your Body: Jump rope is a high-impact activity, and it's important to listen to your body and avoid overtraining. Take breaks as needed, and be mindful of any signs of injury or fatigue.

Building endurance takes time and patience, but with consistent practice and a gradual increase in intensity, you'll be able to improve your endurance and reach your full potential as a jumper.

Improving Coordination

Improving coordination is an important part of jump rope and requires consistent practice and a focus on technique. Here are some tips for improving coordination:

1. Start with Basic Techniques: Mastering the basic techniques of jump rope, such as the basic jump and alternating feet, is the foundation of improving coordination.

2. Focus on Timing: Timing is an important part of jump rope, and involves jumping at the right moment to clear the rope as it swings under your feet. Practice your timing regularly and seek out feedback to improve your coordination.

3. Incorporate Variations: Incorporating different techniques, such as crosses and double unders, into your jump rope routine can help to improve coordination and increase the challenge of your workouts.

4. Practice Regularly: Consistent practice is key to improving coordination. Aim to practice for at least 10-15 minutes each day, gradually increasing the length and intensity of your sessions as you get stronger.

5. Focus on Proper Form: Good technique is key to improving coordination and avoiding injury. Focus on proper form and technique during your workouts, and seek out feedback and tips from more experienced jumpers.

6. Listen to Your Body: Jump rope is a high-impact activity, and it's important to listen to your body

and avoid overtraining. Take breaks as needed, and be mindful of any signs of injury or fatigue.

Improving coordination takes time and patience, but with consistent practice and a focus on technique, you'll be able to improve your coordination and reach your full potential as a jumpe

Strength Training

Strength training is an important part of jump rope and can help to improve your jumping performance and prevent injury. Here are some tips for incorporating strength training into your jump rope routine:

1. Focus on Lower Body: The lower body, including the legs, hips, and core, is the foundation of jump rope and should be the focus of your strength training efforts. Exercises such as squats, lunges, and planks can help to build lower body strength.

2. Incorporate Resistance Training: Resistance training, such as weightlifting, can help to build strength and improve performance. Focus on exercises that target the lower body, such as deadlifts and leg presses.

3. Use Bodyweight Exercises: Bodyweight exercises, such as push-ups, pull-ups, and burpees, can be a convenient and effective way to build strength and improve performance.

4. Incorporate Plyometrics: Plyometric exercises, such as jump squats and box jumps, can help to improve power and explosiveness, which are important components of jump rope.

5. Balance and Stability training: Incorporating balance and stability training into your routine, such as single-leg exercises and balance boards, can help to improve balance and coordination.

6. Gradual Increase: Gradually increase the intensity and weight of your strength training exercises over time, taking care to listen to your body and avoid overtraining.

Strength training is an important part of jump rope and can help to improve your performance and prevent injury. Incorporate strength training into your routine, and you'll soon see the benefits of a stronger and more powerful jump rope performance.

Mental Preparation

Mental preparation is an important part of jump rope and can help to improve focus, reduce stress, and enhance performance. Here are some tips for mental preparation:

1. Set Goals: Set specific, achievable goals for your jump rope training, and use these goals to focus your mind and guide your workouts.

2. Visualize Success: Visualization is a powerful tool that can help you to prepare mentally for your jump rope workouts. Close your eyes and imagine yourself performing at your best, focusing on your technique, timing, and rhythm.

3. Practice Mindfulness: Mindfulness is the practice of being present and focused in the moment. Incorporate mindfulness into your jump rope routine by focusing on your breathing, movements, and sensations as you jump.

4. Manage Stress: Jump rope can be a great stress-reliever, but it's important to manage stress levels in other areas of your life to ensure optimal performance. Incorporate stress-management techniques into your routine, such as meditation, deep breathing, and physical activity.

5. Stay Positive: Maintaining a positive outlook and attitude can help you to overcome challenges and stay motivated. Surround yourself with positive people, and focus on the things you're grateful for, no matter how small.

Mental preparation is an important part of jump rope and can help to improve focus, reduce stress, and enhance performance. By incorporating mental preparation into your routine, you'll be able to jump with confidence and reach your full potential.

Competition and Performance

Competition and performance are exciting aspects of jump rope, and can help to improve skills, challenge yourself, and showcase your talents. Here are some tips for competition and performance:

1. Preparation: Preparation is key to a successful competition or performance. Train consistently, incorporate strength training, and practice visualization and mindfulness to prepare both physically and mentally.

2. Choose the Right Rope: Choosing the right rope is important for competition and performance. Consider factors such as weight, length, and handle grip to ensure optimal performance.

3. Focus on Technique: Good technique is key to a successful competition or performance. Focus on proper form and timing, and seek out feedback and tips from more experienced jumpers.

4. Incorporate Variety: Incorporating different techniques, combinations, and tricks into your performance can help to showcase your skills and make your performance more dynamic and entertaining.

5. Performance Attire: Choose appropriate attire for your performance, such as comfortable and supportive clothing and shoes.

6. Performance Music: Consider incorporating music into your performance to add rhythm and energy

to your jumping. Choose music that you enjoy and that matches the pace and style of your jumping.

Competition and performance are exciting aspects of jump rope that can help you to challenge yourself, showcase your skills, and reach your full potential as a jumper. With preparation and dedication, you'll be able to perform with confidence and enjoy the thrill of competition.

Rules and Regulations

Jump rope competitions have a set of rules and regulations that ensure a fair and safe competition for all participants. Here are some common rules and regulations for jump rope competitions:

1. Age Divisions: Competitions may have different age divisions, such as youth, adult, and senior, to ensure a fair and appropriate competition for all participants.

2. Rope Length: The length of the rope used in competition must meet specific standards, and participants must provide their own rope.

3. Time Limits: Competitions may have time limits for individual and team events, and participants must perform within the specified time frame.

4. Performance Requirements: Participants must perform specific techniques, combinations, and tricks during their performance, and their performance may be judged based on criteria such as timing, rhythm, and execution.

5. Safety: Safety is a top priority in jump rope competitions, and participants must follow all safety guidelines, including wearing appropriate footwear and avoiding dangerous or hazardous movements.

6. Scoring: Participants may be scored based on a set of criteria, such as timing, rhythm, and execution, and scores may be determined by a panel of judges.

Jump rope competitions have specific rules and regulations that ensure a fair and safe competition for all participants. It's important to familiarize yourself with the rules and regulations of the competition you're participating in, and to follow them closely to ensure a successful and enjoyable experience.

Preparing for Competition

Preparing for a jump rope competition requires consistent training, focus, and mental preparation. Here are some tips for preparing for competition:

1. Set Goals: Set specific, achievable goals for your competition, and use these goals to guide your training and focus your mind.

2. Train Consistently: Consistent training is key to preparing for competition. Aim to practice for at least 10-15 minutes each day, gradually increasing the length and intensity of your sessions as you get stronger.

3. Focus on Technique: Good technique is key to a successful competition performance. Focus on proper form and timing, and seek out feedback and tips from more experienced jumpers.

4. Incorporate Strength Training: Strength training, such as weightlifting and plyometrics, can help to improve performance and prevent injury. Incorporate strength training into your routine, and gradually increase the intensity over time.

5. Practice Mental Preparation: Mental preparation, such as visualization and mindfulness, can help to improve focus and reduce stress. Incorporate mental preparation into your routine, and practice visualization and mindfulness regularly.

6. Get Adequate Rest: Adequate rest and recovery are important components of preparing for competition. Get plenty of sleep, and allow your body to recover between training sessions.

Preparing for a jump rope competition requires patience, dedication, and consistency. With these tips, and a focus on training, technique, and mental preparation, you'll be able to perform with confidence and reach your full potential as a jumper.

Performing Under Pressure

Performing under pressure is a common challenge for athletes, including jump ropers. Here are some tips for performing under pressure:

1. Focus on Technique: Good technique is key to a successful performance, and can help to reduce stress and improve confidence under pressure. Focus on proper form and timing, and seek out feedback and tips from more experienced jumpers.

2. Visualize Success: Visualization is a powerful tool that can help you to prepare mentally for your performance. Close your eyes and imagine yourself performing at your best, focusing on your technique, timing, and rhythm.

3. Practice Mindfulness: Mindfulness is the practice of being present and focused in the moment. Incorporate mindfulness into your performance by focusing on your breathing, movements, and sensations as you jump.

4. Manage Stress: Manage stress levels through techniques such as deep breathing, meditation, and physical activity, to ensure optimal performance under pressure.

5. Stay Positive: Maintaining a positive outlook and attitude can help you to overcome challenges and stay motivated. Surround yourself with positive people, and focus on the things you're grateful for, no matter how small.

6. Rehearse: Rehearse your performance in similar conditions as the competition, such as with an audience or with background noise, to help you get used to performing under pressure.

Performing under pressure can be challenging, but with preparation and focus, you'll be able to perform with confidence and reach your full potential as a jumper. Remember, the most important thing is to have fun and enjoy the process!

Tips for Success

Jump rope is a fun and challenging activity that requires dedication, consistency, and a focus on technique. Here are some tips for success:

1. Start Slow: Start with short jump rope sessions and gradually increase the length and intensity of your workouts as you get stronger.

2. Focus on Technique: Good technique is key to success and avoiding injury. Focus on proper form and timing, and seek out feedback and tips from more experienced jumpers.

3. Incorporate Strength Training: Strength training, such as weightlifting and plyometrics, can help to improve performance and prevent injury. Incorporate strength training into your routine, and gradually increase the intensity over time.

4. Practice Mental Preparation: Mental preparation, such as visualization and mindfulness, can help to improve focus and reduce stress. Incorporate mental preparation into your routine, and practice visualization and mindfulness regularly.

5. Set Goals: Set specific, achievable goals for your jump rope training, and use these goals to guide your workouts and track your progress.

6. Listen to Your Body: Jump rope is a high-impact activity, and it's important to listen to your body and avoid overtraining. Take breaks as needed, and be mindful of any signs of injury or fatigue.

With dedication, consistency, and a focus on technique, you'll be able to reach your full potential as a jumper and

enjoy the many benefits of this fun and challenging
activity.

Conclusion

In conclusion, jump rope is a fun and challenging activity that offers numerous physical and mental benefits. With its roots dating back to ancient civilizations, jump rope has evolved into a popular and competitive sport that requires dedication, consistency, and a focus on technique. Whether you're looking to improve your fitness, build strength, or perform in competitions, jump rope can help you to reach your goals. By following the tips and guidelines outlined in this book, you'll be able to get started with jump rope, improve your skills, and reach your full potential as a jumper. So grab a rope, and start skipping today!

Reflections on the Journey

Jump rope is a journey, and like any journey, it's a chance to reflect on progress, growth, and the lessons learned along the way. Here are some reflections on the journey of jump rope:

1. Remember Your Beginnings: Take a moment to reflect on your first steps with jump rope and remember how far you've come since then. Celebrate your progress and the achievements you've made along the way.

2. Recognize Your Growth: Jump rope is a journey of growth and improvement, both physically and mentally. Take a moment to recognize the growth you've made in your skills, strength, and mental preparation.

3. Embrace the Process: Jump rope is a process, and it's important to embrace the ups and downs along the way. Embrace the challenges and setbacks as opportunities to grow and improve, and celebrate each small victory along the way.

4. Reflect on Lessons Learned: Jump rope is a journey of learning, and it's important to reflect on the lessons learned along the way. Take a moment to reflect on the tips and techniques you've learned, and how they've helped you to improve your skills and reach your goals.

5. Look Ahead: Jump rope is a journey that never truly ends, and it's important to look ahead to the future and set new goals for your continued growth and improvement.

Jump rope is a journey of growth, improvement, and discovery, and it's important to reflect on the progress made along the way. Embrace the process, celebrate your achievements, and look ahead to the future, and you'll be able to reach your full potential as a jumper.

Inspiring Stories from Top Jumpers

Jump rope is a sport that has inspired many athletes to reach their full potential and achieve greatness. Here are some inspiring stories from top jumpers:

1. Buddy Lee: Buddy Lee is a former US Army jump rope champion and is widely considered to be one of the greatest jump rope athletes of all time. He has won numerous national and world championships, and is a sought-after motivational speaker and coach.

2. Karen Hardy: Karen Hardy is a former US national jump rope champion who has used her skills and passion for jump rope to inspire others and promote the sport. She has performed in numerous competitions and exhibitions, and is a sought-after coach and instructor.

3. Tim Furgeson: Tim Furgeson is a former US national jump rope champion and world record holder who has inspired countless others with his dedication and passion for the sport. He has competed in numerous international competitions and exhibitions, and is a sought-after coach and instructor.

4. Johnny "Jump Rope" Diggs: Johnny Diggs is a former US national jump rope champion who has used his skills and passion for jump rope to inspire others and promote the sport. He has performed in numerous competitions and exhibitions, and is a sought-after coach and instructor.

These top jumpers are proof that with dedication, hard work, and a passion for the sport, anyone can reach their full potential as a jumper and achieve greatness. Their inspiring stories serve as a reminder that anything is possible with the right mindset and approach.

Final Thoughts and Encouragement

Jump rope is a fun, challenging, and rewarding activity that offers numerous physical and mental benefits. Whether you're just starting out or looking to improve your skills, the journey of jump rope is one of growth, improvement, and discovery. Remember to embrace the process, celebrate your achievements, and set new goals for your continued growth and improvement. Above all, have fun and enjoy the journey!

To all aspiring jumpers, never give up on your dreams and always believe in yourself. With dedication, consistency, and a focus on technique, you'll be able to reach your full potential and achieve greatness. So grab a rope, and start skipping today!

Glossary of Terms

1. Rope: A piece of equipment used for jumping, typically made of plastic or leather and ranging in length from 7-9 feet.

2. Timing: The rhythm and pace of jumping, which is key to a successful performance.

3. Double Under: A jump rope technique in which the rope passes under the feet twice with a single jump.

4. Crosses: A jump rope technique in which the rope crosses in front of the body.

5. Speed Skipping: A jump rope technique that involves jumping at a fast pace.

6. Tricks and Combinations: Complex jump rope techniques that involve a combination of basic and advanced techniques, often performed in a creative and entertaining manner.

7. Endurance: The ability to sustain physical activity for an extended period of time.

8. Coordination: The ability to coordinate movements effectively and efficiently.

9. Strength Training: Physical exercise that focuses on building strength and muscle mass.

10. Mental Preparation: The process of preparing mentally for physical activity, often through visualization and mindfulness.

11. Competition: A competitive event in which
participants perform jump rope techniques and are
judged based on specific criteria.

12. Performance: A showcase of jump rope skills,
often performed in front of an audience.

This glossary of terms provides a basic understanding of
the language and concepts commonly used in jump rope,
and is a useful resource for anyone looking to get started
or improve their skills in this exciting and challenging sport.